"THE MIRACULOUS WORLD OF MIRACLE BERRIES"

Unleashing Nature's Sweet Secret

@Copyright (2023) by R. Vilar – All rights reserved.

The content of the book may not be reproduced, duplicated or transmitted without direct written permission from the author. Under no circumstances will any legal responsibility or blame be held against the publisher for any reparation, damages, or monetary loss due to the information herein, either directly or indirectly.

Legal Notice

This book is copyright protected. This is only for personal use. You cannot amend, distribute, sell, use quote or paraphrase any part or the content within the book without the consent of the author.

ISBN: 9798398578881

Published by: Greener Planet 4us Ltd.

Disclaimer Notice:

Please note the information contained within the document is for educational and entertainment purpose only. Every attempt has been made to provide accurate, up to date and reliable complete information. No warranties of any kind are expressed or implied. Readers acknowledge that the author is not engaged in the rendering of legal, financial, medical or professional advice. The content of this book has been derived from various sources, Please consult a licenced professional before attempting any techniques outlined in this book.

By reading this document, the reader agrees that under no circumstances is the author responsible for any losses, direct or indirect, which are incurred a result of the use of the information contained within the document, including but not limited to, - errors, omissions, or inaccuracies

CONTENTS

- INTRODUCTION 7
- **CHAPTER 1** 9
  - INTRODUCTION TO MIRACLE BERRIES 9
  - DEFINITION OF MIRACLE BERRIES 9
  - HISTORY AND CULTURAL SIGNIFICANCE: 10
  - MAIN THEMES AND TOPICS COVERED IN THE BOOK: 10
  - CONCLUSION 11
- **CHAPTER 2** 13
  - THE HISTORY AND DISCOVERY OF MIRACLE BERRIES 13
  - ORIGIN AND EARLY USE OF MIRACLE BERRIES 13
  - STORIES AND ANECDOTES OF MIRACLE BERRIES FROM AROUND THE WORLD 14
  - HISTORICAL REFERENCES TO MIRACLE BERRIES IN LITERATURE, FOLKLORE, AND CULINARY TRADITIONS 15
  - CONCLUSION 15
- **CHAPTER 3** 17
  - THE SCIENCE OF MIRACLE BERRIES 17
  - BOTANICAL CHARACTERISTICS AND SCIENTIFIC CLASSIFICATION OF MIRACLE BERRIES 17
  - BIOACTIVE COMPOUNDS IN MIRACLE BERRIES 18
  - PHYSIOLOGICAL AND BIOCHEMICAL MECHANISMS OF THE MIRACLE BERRY PHENOMENON 19
  - CONCLUSION 20
- **CHAPTER 4** 23
  - CULTIVATING MIRACLE BERRIES 23
  - SPECIES AND VARIETIES OF MIRACLE BERRIES 23
  - NATIVE HABITATS AND GROWING REQUIREMENTS 24
  - PROPAGATION TECHNIQUES 24

CHALLENGES AND CONSIDERATIONS IN GROWING MIRACLE BERRIES 25

HARVESTING, PROCESSING, AND PRESERVING MIRACLE BERRIES 25

BEST PRACTICES FOR CULTIVATING MIRACLE BERRIES 27

CONCLUSION 28

CHAPTER 5 29

CULINARY ALCHEMY: EXPERIMENTING WITH MIRACLE BERRIES IN THE KITCHEN 29

CONCLUSION 34

CHAPTER 6 37

THE SWEET SIDE OF HEALTH: NUTRITIONAL BENEFITS OF MIRACLE BERRIES 37

ROLE OF MIRACLE BERRIES IN MANAGING TASTE-RELATED CHALLENGES 38

POTENTIAL HEALTH BENEFITS OF MIRACLE BERRIES 39

LIMITATIONS AND NEED FOR FURTHER RESEARCH ON MIRACLE BERRIES 44

CHAPTER 7 47

EXPLORING FLAVOUR PERCEPTION: HOW MIRACLE BERRIES CHALLENGE OUR TASTE BUDS 47

CHAPTER 8 53

BEYOND THE TASTE: OTHER USES AND APPLICATIONS OF MIRACLE BERRIES 53

NON-CULINARY APPLICATIONS OF MIRACLE BERRIES 53

HISTORICAL AND CONTEMPORARY USES OF MIRACLE BERRIES 55

POTENTIAL FUTURE DEVELOPMENTS AND APPLICATIONS 56

CHAPTER 9 59

FROM SCIENCE TO SENSATION: STORIES AND EXPERIENCES OF MIRACLE BERRY ENTHUSIASTS 59

REAL-LIFE STORIES OF HOW MIRACLE BERRIES HAVE IMPACTED PEOPLE'S PERCEPTION OF TASTE AND FLAVOUR .. 59

INSIGHTS FROM CHEFS, FOOD SCIENTISTS, AND OTHER EXPERTS ON THEIR EXPERIENCES WITH MIRACLE BERRIES .. 60

PERSONAL ANECDOTES AND TESTIMONIALS FROM MIRACLE BERRY ENTHUSIASTS 61

CONCLUSION 61

CHAPTER 10 63

THE FUTURE OF MIRACLE BERRIES: UNLEASHING THE FULL POTENTIAL OF NATURE'S SWEET SECRET 63

SUMMARIZING THE CURRENT STATE OF RESEARCH AND KNOWLEDGE ON MIRACLE BERRIES 63

POTENTIAL FUTURE DEVELOPMENTS AND APPLICATIONS OF MIRACLE BERRIES 64

SPECULATING ON THE POSSIBILITIES AND CHALLENGES OF HARNESSING THE FULL POTENTIAL OF NATURE'S SWEET SECRET 66

CONCLUSION 68

BONUS!!! 69

30 RECIPES THAT UTILIZE MIRACLE BERRIES 69

10 COCKTAILS RECIPES USING MIRACLE BERRIES 74

10 DESSERT RECIPES THAT INCORPORATE MIRACLE BERRIES TO CREATE UNIQUE AND SWEET TREATS: 76

REFERENCES 80

Introduction

Unleash the Sweet Secret of Nature's Miracle Berries

Welcome to "The Miraculous World of Miracle Berries: Unleashing Nature's Sweet Secret"! Are you ready to embark on a captivating journey into the realm of taste-altering wonders? If you've ever been intrigued by the idea of a berry that can transform sour into sweet, unlock hidden flavors, and challenge your taste buds, then this book is for you.

In these pages, we will unravel the fascinating story of miracle berries and delve into their rich history, remarkable properties, and endless possibilities. Whether you're a food enthusiast, a health-conscious individual, or simply curious about the wonders of nature, this book will leave you amazed and inspired.

Why should you read this book? The answer lies in the allure and potential of miracle berries. These small, unassuming fruits hold within them the power to change how we perceive taste. Imagine biting into a lemon and experiencing a burst of sweet citrus instead of puckering sourness. Envision savoring a bowl of tart yogurt that magically becomes a delectable dessert. With miracle berries, the ordinary becomes extraordinary, and the mundane becomes a culinary adventure.

But this book is not just about the taste-altering effects of miracle berries. It goes beyond that. We will explore the science behind these berries, unraveling the mysteries of their unique properties and the physiological mechanisms that make them so remarkable. We will dive into the world of cultivation, learning how to grow and harvest these precious berries to enjoy their flavors at home. And we will venture into the realm of nutrition and health, discovering the potential benefits of incorporating miracle berries into our diets.

"The Miraculous World of Miracle Berries" is not just a collection of scientific facts and culinary experiments. It is a celebration of nature's ingenuity, a tribute to the endless possibilities that lie within the realm of our senses. By understanding and harnessing the power of miracle berries, we can transform our perception of taste, explore new dimensions of flavor, and even improve our relationship with food.

So, whether you're a food lover seeking new culinary adventures, a health enthusiast looking for natural alternatives, or simply someone curious about the wonders of the natural world, this book invites you to open your mind, tantalize your taste buds, and embrace the sweetness that awaits.

Join me on this extraordinary journey through "The Miraculous World of Miracle Berries: Unleashing Nature's Sweet Secret." Let's unlock the hidden flavors and uncover the secrets of these remarkable berries together.

CHAPTER 1

INTRODUCTION TO MIRACLE BERRIES

Miracle berries are a remarkable fruit that has gained widespread attention due to their unique taste-altering properties. Have you heard of miracle berries? They're an exciting fruit that has become quite popular because they can change the way things taste! In this chapter, we'll explore what miracle berries are, their history, and why they're important. We'll also give you an idea of what you can expect to learn about in the rest of the book.

DEFINITION OF MIRACLE BERRIES

Miracle berries come from West Africa and are small red fruit. Their scientific name is Synsepalum dulcificum. When you eat them alone, they taste slightly sweet and are about the same size as a coffee bean. Miracle berries are unique because they have the ability to change the way things taste when you eat them.

The unique taste-altering properties of miracle berries are attributed to a protein called miraculin, which is found in the fruit. Eating something containing miraculin protein interacts with your taste buds and changes how they respond to different tastes. This makes sour and bitter flavors taste sweet instead. This remarkable phenomenon has fascinated scientists, chefs, and food enthusiasts alike, leading to the exploration of various culinary applications of miracle berries.

HISTORY AND CULTURAL SIGNIFICANCE:

The history of miracle berries dates back centuries in West Africa, where local tribes have used them for their taste-modifying properties and medicinal benefits. The use of miracle berries in traditional culinary practices, medicinal remedies, and cultural rituals has been an integral part of the heritage and traditions of certain tribes in West Africa.

In recent times, miracle berries have become culturally significant, especially in the culinary industry. People who love food, such as chefs, mixologists, and food enthusiasts worldwide, have been fascinated by the special qualities of miracle berries. They use them in their cooking and drinks to make new, unique, and unforgettable dining experiences. The growing popularity of miracle berries has also led to the emergence of niche markets and industries centered around these fascinating fruits.

MAIN THEMES AND TOPICS COVERED IN THE BOOK:

In this book, we will look at many different things about miracle berries, such as how they change the way things taste, how they were used in the past, how they are used in current cooking, how they might help your health and more. Some of the important ideas and topics that this book talks about are:

- Science of Miracle Berries: We will delve into the scientific aspects of miracle berries, including the composition of miraculin, the taste-modifying mechanism, and the latest research findings in the field of taste perception.

- Traditional Uses: We will explore the historical and cultural significance of miracle berries in West African communities, including their conventional culinary, medicinal, and ritualistic uses.
- Culinary Applications: We will look into the modern-day culinary applications of miracle berries, including their use in food and beverage pairings, flavor transformations, and creative culinary experiments.
- Health Benefits: We will examine the potential health benefits of miracle berries, including their antioxidant properties, potential impact on blood sugar levels, and other potential health effects.
- Practical Tips and Recipes: We will provide practical tips on using and incorporating miracle berries into culinary creations and recipes and ideas for experimenting with these unique fruits in the kitchen.
- Future Possibilities: We will explore the potential future applications of miracle berries, including their use in the food industry, potential therapeutic uses, and emerging trends related to these fascinating fruits.

CONCLUSION

Miracle berries are a strange food that has gotten people all over the world interested and thinking. In this section, we talked about what wonder berries are, how they came to be, and what they mean to different tribes. We also gave an outline of the main themes and topics covered in this book. In the next chapters, we'll learn more about the mysterious world of wonder berries, and also find out their secrets, and look at different ways they can be used.

CHAPTER 2

THE HISTORY AND DISCOVERY OF MIRACLE BERRIES

Miracle berries have a captivating history that spans continents and time periods, with tales of their discovery and historical uses intriguingly diverse. In this chapter, we will explore the origin and early use of miracle berries, including their discovery by Western explorers in West Africa in the 18th century. We will also find stories and tales from all over the world about how miracle berries were found and used in the past, as well as references to them in literature, folklore, and food traditions, which will show off their rich cultural history.

ORIGIN AND EARLY USE OF MIRACLE BERRIES

Miracle berries are believed to have originated in West Africa, particularly in countries such as Ghana, Nigeria, and Cameroon. Local groups in these regions have used them for a long time because of how they change the way things taste. They have known this for generations.

Western explorers' earliest documented encounter with miracle berries dates back to the 18th century. In 1725, a French explorer named Chevalier des Marchais first reported the existence of a "miraculous fruit" during his travels in West Africa. He described how the berry, when consumed, could make sour or acidic foods taste sweet, and this property fascinated him.

However, it wasn't until the 19th century that more detailed accounts of miracle berries began to emerge, with explorers and botanists documenting their properties and uses. In 1852, a British explorer named Richard Francis Burton encountered miracle berries during his travels in West Africa and documented their effects in his writings. This sparked further interest among botanists and explorers, and more reports of the unique taste-modifying properties of miracle berries began to surface.

STORIES AND ANECDOTES OF MIRACLE BERRIES FROM AROUND THE WORLD

Miracle berries have always intrigued people from different countries and time periods, leading to many interesting stories about how they were found and used in the past.

For instance, there are accounts of how local tribes in West Africa have traditionally used miracle berries to enhance the taste of their food and make sour or bitter foods more palatable. They would chew on the berries or use their juice to coat their tongues before consuming other foods, transforming the taste experience.

In Japan, miracle berries are known as "mirakuru na kajitsu" and have become a novelty item in culinary experiences. There are tales of how people in Japan have hosted "flavor tripping" parties, where guests consume miracle berries and then enjoy an array of sour or bitter foods that are transformed into sweet delights. This trend has gained traction in recent years, with restaurants and culinary enthusiasts incorporating miracle berries into unique dining experiences.

HISTORICAL REFERENCES TO MIRACLE BERRIES IN LITERATURE, FOLKLORE, AND CULINARY TRADITIONS

Miracle berries have also found their way into various cultures' literature, folklore, and culinary traditions, showcasing their cultural significance and heritage.

For example, there are references to miracle berries in traditional African folklore, where they are believed to possess mystical powers and are used in rituals or as offerings to deities. Some African communities use miracle berries in cultural ceremonies or celebrations to mark special occasions, believing in their magical and transformative properties.

In literature, miracle berries have been mentioned in travelogues, culinary writings, and other literary works, describing their unique properties and uses. There are also references to miracle berries in historical cookbooks, where they are used as a natural sweetener or flavor enhancer in various culinary preparations. Throughout history, people have been fascinated by the magical properties of berries, as evidenced by various literary and culinary examples. These examples also demonstrate how berries can be used in cooking.

CONCLUSION

We have looked into the origin and early usage of miracle berries in West Africa, as well as tales and anecdotes from all over the globe, as well as allusions to miracle berries in literature, folklore, and culinary traditions. The rich cultural heritage of miracle berries highlights their long-standing significance and fascination among different cultures and time periods. In the following chapters, we will continue our journey into the world of miracle berries, uncovering more secrets and unraveling their intriguing history.

CHAPTER 3

THE SCIENCE OF MIRACLE BERRIES

Miracle berries, scientifically known as Synsepalum dulcificum, are a unique fruit that has garnered attention for their taste-modifying properties. This chapter will look in-depth at the botanical characteristics and scientific classification of miracle berries, including their plant anatomy, growth patterns, and reproductive mechanisms. We will also explore the bioactive compounds responsible for the taste-modifying effects of miracle berries, such as miraculin and other glycoproteins, and delve into the physiological and biochemical mechanisms behind the miracle berry phenomenon, including the interactions with taste receptors on the tongue and the molecular events that lead to the perception of sweetness.

BOTANICAL CHARACTERISTICS AND SCIENTIFIC CLASSIFICATION OF MIRACLE BERRIES

Miracle berries are small red berries that are native to West Africa and belong to the Sapotaceae family. These tropical and subtropical fruits are typically found growing on evergreen shrubs or small trees that can reach heights of up to 5 meters. The leaves of miracle berry plants are elliptical and leathery, with a glossy appearance, and they are arranged alternately on the stems. The flowers of miracle berry plants are small and white, and they are usually inconspicuous.

Miracle berry plants are adapted to well-drained, acidic soils and are known to be slow-growing plants that can take several years to reach maturity and produce fruit. They are typically propagated through seeds, cuttings, or grafting. The plants are susceptible to cold and strong temperature swings, and they thrive when kept warm and wet.

BIOACTIVE COMPOUNDS IN MIRACLE BERRIES

The taste-modifying properties of miracle berries can be attributed to their bioactive compounds, with miraculin being the most well-known and extensively studied. Miraculin is a glycoprotein that is found in the pulp of miracle berries and is responsible for the phenomenon of taste alteration.

Miraculin works by attaching itself to the taste receptors on the tongue that are in charge of identifying sour or acidic tastes. This binding alters the shape and function of the taste receptors, causing them to perceive sour or acidic tastes as sweet. This molecular interaction between miraculin and taste receptors leads to the remarkable taste-modifying effects of miracle berries, where sour or acidic foods are transformed into sweet-tasting delights.

Apart from miraculin, miracle berries have other glycoproteins and bioactive compounds that play a role in altering their taste. Some of these compounds are still being studied, and their exact mechanisms of action are not yet fully understood. However, research suggests that these compounds synergize with miraculin to create the unique taste experience associated with miracle berries.

PHYSIOLOGICAL AND BIOCHEMICAL MECHANISMS OF THE MIRACLE BERRY PHENOMENON

The taste-modifying effects of miracle berries involve complex physiological and biochemical mechanisms. When a person consumes a miracle berry, the miraculin in the berry interacts with the taste receptors on the tongue, leading to a series of molecular events that result in the perception of sweetness.

When miraculin binds to the taste receptors responsible for detecting sour or acidic flavors, it triggers a cascade of biochemical reactions within the taste buds. This cascade of events leads to the activation of intracellular signaling pathways and the release of neurotransmitters, ultimately resulting in the perception of sweetness, even in the absence of actual sugar or sweet compounds.

Furthermore, research suggests that the taste-modifying effects of miracle berries may also involve interactions with other sensory receptors in the mouth, such as those responsible for detecting temperature and texture. For example, miraculin has been found to enhance the perception of sweetness in foods with certain textures, such as creamy or fatty textures, further adding to the complexity of the miracle berry phenomenon.

Further, it's important to remember that the impact of miraculin may differ from person to person based on their genetic composition and the particular taste receptors found on their tongue. Different people may perceive sweetness differently. Some may find it more intense, while others may find it less noticeable. This shows how genetics, biochemistry, and taste perception are all connected when it comes to miracle berries.

Scientists are still studying how miracle berries work on a physiological and biochemical level. They are discovering new information about how the bioactive compounds in miracle berries, like miraculin, interact with taste and sensory receptors in the mouth to create their unique taste-modifying effects.

CONCLUSION

In conclusion, the taste-modifying properties of miracle berries can be attributed to their bioactive compounds, primarily miraculin and other glycoproteins. These compounds interact with taste receptors on the tongue, triggering molecular events that lead to the perception of sweetness, even without actual sugar or sweet compounds. The physiological and biochemical mechanisms behind the miracle berry phenomenon are complex and involve interactions with taste receptors, intracellular signaling pathways, and other sensory receptors in the mouth.

The scientific exploration of miracle berries and their taste-modifying effects provides fascinating insights into the intricate mechanisms of taste perception and the interplay between bioactive compounds, genetics, and sensory receptors. Further research in this area may have potential applications in various fields, such as food science, nutrition, and medicine. It could lead to the development of novel taste-modifying agents or therapeutic interventions for individuals with altered taste perception due to medical conditions or other factors.

The taste-modifying properties of these substances, along with their unique botanical and biochemical characteristics, are quite fascinating. Miracle berries continue to capture the curiosity of researchers, food enthusiasts, and consumers alike, offering a unique and enjoyable sensory experience that challenges our understanding of taste perception and the science of flavours.

CHAPTER 4

CULTIVATING MIRACLE BERRIES

Miracle berries, with their unique taste-modifying properties, have gained popularity among food enthusiasts, culinary professionals, and home gardenersIn this chapter, we'll explore the intricacies of producing miracle berries, from the numerous species and types available to details on their ideal growing conditions, propagation methods, and harvesting and storing strategies.

SPECIES AND VARIETIES OF MIRACLE BERRIES

Miracle berries belong to the Synsepalum genus within the Sapotaceae family and are primarily represented by two main species: Synsepalum dulcificum, also known as the classic miracle berry, and Synsepalum kilimandscharicum, commonly referred to as the Tanzanian miracle berry. These species are native to West Africa and East Africa and have slightly different botanical characteristics, growth habits, and flavor profiles.

Apart from the two main species, other Synsepalum species share similar taste-modifying properties, albeit to a lesser extent. These include Synsepalum subcordatum, Synsepalum brevipes, and Synsepalum cerasiferum, among others. Some enthusiasts also cultivate these lesser-known species for their unique taste-altering effects.

NATIVE HABITATS AND GROWING REQUIREMENTS

Miracle berries are typically found in tropical and subtropical regions of Africa, where they grow in the wild under specific environmental conditions. Understanding the native habitats and growing requirements of miracle berries is crucial for successful cultivation.

Miracle berries prefer well-draining, slightly acidic to neutral soils with good organic matter content. They thrive in a warm and humid climate, with temperatures ranging from 60 to 85°F (15 to 30°C). They require filtered sunlight or partial shade, as excessive direct sunlight can damage delicate leaves and fruits. Adequate moisture, through regular watering or rainfall, is essential to keep the plants healthy and to promote flowering and fruiting.

PROPAGATION TECHNIQUES

Multiple methods, including seeding, cuttings, and grafting, exist for the propagation of miracle berries. The most popular way of propagation is seeds, which must be germinated in ideal circumstances like moderate temperatures, high humidity, and well-drained soil. Cuttings can also be taken from mature plants and rooted in a suitable medium, but this method can be challenging due to the delicate nature of miracle berry plants.

Miracle berries may also be propagated by grafting, preferably onto the rootstock of an acceptable fruit tree or a member of a closely related species. The grafted plants gain from the established root system of the rootstock, allowing for faster and more consistent results.

CHALLENGES AND CONSIDERATIONS IN GROWING MIRACLE BERRIES

Cultivating miracle berries can pose some challenges and considerations, particularly for those outside their native regions. One of the main challenges is creating optimal growing conditions, including providing the right temperature, humidity, light, and soil conditions. Miracle berries are sensitive to extreme temperatures, excessive sunlight, and overly wet or dry conditions, which can affect their growth and fruiting.

Another consideration is the availability and quality of seeds or plant materials. Sourcing reliable and authentic miracle berry seeds or plants can be crucial for successful cultivation. Additionally, since miracle berries are still relatively uncommon, finding technical information and resources on their cultivation may require some research and effort.

HARVESTING, PROCESSING, AND PRESERVING MIRACLE BERRIES

Harvesting miracle berries at the right stage of ripeness is essential for optimal flavor and taste-modifying effects. The fruits should be fully matured, with a deep red or purple color and a slightly soft texture. They can be gently plucked from the plant, taking care not to damage the delicate skin.

Miracle berries may be processed and conserved in a number of ways to increase their storage life and keep their flavor-altering qualities intact. Best practices include the following:

1. Fresh Consumption:

Fresh miracle berries can be consumed immediately after harvesting. Simply rinse the berries in clean water and remove the seeds, if desired. The fruit can be eaten on its own or used to alter the taste of other foods and beverages.

2. Drying:

Miracle berries can be dried for longer-term storage. After rinsing and removing the seeds, place the berries on a clean paper towel or a drying rack in a well-ventilated area. Allow them to air dry for several days until they are fully dehydrated, with a leathery texture. Once dried, the berries can be stored in an airtight container in a cool, dry place.

3. Freezing:

Another way to preserve miracle berries is by freezing them. After rinsing and removing the seeds, place the berries in a single layer on a baking sheet or a plate, and freeze them for a few hours until they are firm. The berries may be frozen for up to several months after being transferred to an airtight container or freezer bag. Frozen miracle berries can be thawed before use or used directly in frozen desserts or beverages.

4. Canning or Jam Making:

Miracle berries can be preserved through canning or by making jams. First, rinse the berries and remove the seeds. Then, put them in a saucepan with sugar or your preferred sweetener. Simmer the mixture gently until the berries soften, and their juices are released. Next, you'll want to move the berries and juice into jars that have been sterilized. Then, follow the correct canning procedures to process them. You can also make jam by mashing the cooked berries and adding sugar. After that, you can store the jam in sterilized jars in the refrigerator or freezer.

BEST PRACTICES FOR CULTIVATING MIRACLE BERRIES

To successfully cultivate miracle berries, consider the following best practices:

1. Choosing the right species or variety of miracle berries for your climate and growing conditions. Synsepalum dulcificum is more commonly cultivated and tends to be more adaptable to different environments, while Synsepalum kilimandscharicum is more challenging to grow and requires specific conditions.
2. Provide the optimal growing conditions, including well-draining, slightly acidic to neutral soil, warm and humid climate, filtered sunlight or partial shade, and regular watering or rainfall.
3. Propagate miracle berries using suitable methods such as seeds, cuttings, or grafting, considering each method's specific requirements and challenges.
4. Take care of the delicate nature of miracle berry plants, including protecting them from extreme temperatures, excessive sunlight, and overly wet or dry conditions.
5. Harvest the berries at the right stage of ripeness for optimal flavor and taste-modifying effects.
6. Process and preserve miracle berries using suitable drying, freezing, canning, or jam-making methods to extend their shelf-life and retain their taste-modifying properties.

CONCLUSION

Cultivating miracle berries can be a rewarding and enjoyable endeavor for those interested in exploring their unique taste-modifying effects. Understanding the different species and varieties, native habitats, growing requirements, propagation techniques, and best practices for harvesting, processing, and preserving miracle berries can help ensure successful cultivation. With proper care and attention, you can enjoy the wonder of these remarkable plants and experiment with their taste-altering properties in your culinary adventures.

CHAPTER 5

CULINARY ALCHEMY: EXPERIMENTING WITH MIRACLE BERRIES IN THE KITCHEN

With their unique taste-modifying effects, Miracle berries offer an exciting opportunity for culinary experimentation in the kitchen. In this chapter, we will delve into the diverse culinary applications of miracle berries and explore how they can be used to enhance flavors, create flavor illusions, experiment with culinary combinations, and incorporate them into everyday meals, special occasions, and even molecular gastronomy.

Enhancing Flavours

One of the fascinating aspects of miracle berries is their ability to transform sour or acidic flavors into sweetness. When consumed after consuming miracle berries, sour foods like citrus fruits, vinegar, or yogurt can taste surprisingly sweet, offering a delightful sensory experience. The natural sweetness of fruits can also be enhanced when paired with miracle berries, intensifying their flavors and making them even more enjoyable.

To experiment with enhancing flavors using miracle berries, you can try making a citrus fruit salad with lemon, lime, and grapefruit and consume it after consuming miracle berries. You'll be pleasantly surprised by how the once tangy and sour flavors transform into a burst of natural sweetness on your taste buds.

Flavor Illusions

Miracle berries can create flavor illusions by making foods taste completely different from what we expect. For example, traditionally bitter foods like dark chocolate, coffee, or Brussels sprouts can taste sweet and enjoyable after consuming miracle berries. This opens up a whole new world of possibilities for experimenting with different flavor combinations and creating unique taste sensations.

To experiment with flavor illusions, you can try tasting a piece of dark chocolate or drinking a cup of black coffee before and after consuming miracle berries. Notice how the flavors transform from bitter to sweet, offering a surprising and delightful sensory experience.

Culinary Combinations

Miracle berries are a great way to experiment with new and exciting flavor combinations in your cooking. By pairing them with savory or bitter foods, you can create a unique and delicious taste that perfectly complements the other flavors. For example, pairing miracle berries with cheese, pickles, or olives can transform the normally sour or bitter flavors into sweetness, creating a unique and unexpected taste sensation.

To experiment with culinary combinations, you can try making a cheese platter with different types of cheese, including some sour or bitter options, and consume it after consuming miracle berries. Notice how the flavors of the cheese are transformed into sweetness, creating a unique and delightful culinary experience.

Recipes and Cooking Techniques

There are many recipes and cooking methods that can show how miracle berries can change the way food tastes. For instance, you can use miracle berries to make a sorbet or granita with sour fruits like lemons or limes, making a dessert that is both sweet and spicy. To add a twist to your drinks, try mixing cocktails, mocktails, or infused waters using miracle berries.

Making a lemon or lime sorbet by mixing the fruit juice with little water and sweetening it with miracle berries is a fun way to experiment with new flavors and cooking methods. Put the mixture in the freezer, and then serve it as a sweet and sour treat.

Everyday Meals and Special Occasions

Miracle berries can be incorporated into everyday meals and special occasions to elevate the dining experience. For example, you can use them in sauces, dressings, marinades, or glazes to add a touch of sweetness to savory dishes like grilled chicken, roasted vegetables, or seafood. You can also use them in desserts, baked goods, or confections to reduce the need for added sugar while still enjoying a sweet taste.

To incorporate miracle berries into everyday meals, you can try making a tangy-sweet marinade for the chicken by blending lemon juice, olive oil, garlic, herbs, and some powdered miracle berries. Marinate the chicken for a few hours, then grill or roast it for a delicious and unique flavor profile.

You can use miracle berries for special occasions to create a memorable and interactive dining experience. Set up a tasting station with a variety of sour or bitter foods, such as citrus fruits, pickles, vinegar, or bitter greens, along with some powdered miracle berries. Encourage your guests to try the foods before and after consuming miracle berries and watch as their taste buds are amazed by the transformation of flavors.

Molecular Gastronomy

Miracle berries have also found their way into the world of molecular gastronomy, where chefs and food scientists use them to create innovative and avant-garde culinary creations. Miracle berries can be used to manipulate flavors, textures, and taste perceptions in molecular gastronomy techniques such as spherification, foam-making, or encapsulation, resulting in visually stunning and creative unique dishes.

To experiment with molecular gastronomy using miracle berries, make a citrus fruit caviar by mixing fruit juice with sodium alginate and then drop the mixture into a calcium chloride solution to form gelatinous spheres. Serve the citrus caviar on a spoon and have your guests consume a miracle berry before tasting the caviar. Watch as their taste buds are fooled by the intense sweetness of the once-sour citrus caviar.

Health Benefits

Besides their culinary applications, miracle berries offer potential health benefits. They are low in calories, naturally sweet, and can be used as a sugar substitute in certain recipes, making them suitable for those watching their sugar intake or managing diabetes. Miracle berries are also rich in antioxidants, fiber, and other beneficial compounds that can support overall health and well-being.

However, it's important to note that while miracle berries can enhance the taste of sour or bitter foods, they should not replace a healthy and balanced diet. Moderation is key, and it's best to consult with a healthcare professional before making any significant dietary changes or using miracle berries for health purposes.

Safety Considerations

Even though miracle berries are usually thought to be safe to eat, there are a few things to keep in mind. Some people may have allergic responses or stomach problems after eating miracle berries, but this isn't very common. It's also important to know that miracle berries can briefly change how people taste things, which can make some foods or drinks less enjoyable.

It's best to start with a small amount of miracle berries and gradually raise it as needed. If you have any bad responses, you should stop eating them. If you already have a health problem or worry about your health, it's best to talk to a doctor before eating miracle berries.

Sourcing and Storage

Miracle berries can be found in various forms, including fresh berries, freeze-dried berries, or powdered berries. Fresh miracle berries are typically the most potent in terms of taste-modifying effects, but they are also more perishable and can be harder to find. Freeze-dried or powdered miracle berries are more readily available and have a longer shelf life, but their taste-modifying effects may be less intense.

When sourcing miracle berries, choosing a reputable supplier is important to ensure quality and safety. Store miracle berries according to the manufacturer's instructions and keep them in a cool, dry place away from direct sunlight to preserve their potency.

CONCLUSION

Miracle berries are a unique and fascinating ingredient that can add an element of culinary alchemy to your kitchen experiments. From enhancing flavors and creating flavor illusions to experimenting with culinary combinations, incorporating miracle berries into recipes and cooking techniques, using them in everyday meals and special occasions, exploring molecular gastronomy, and considering their potential health benefits and safety considerations, there are endless possibilities for culinary creativity with miracle berries.

Whether you're a home cook, a professional chef, or simply a food enthusiast, experimenting with miracle berries can be a fun and exciting culinary adventure. As with any new ingredient, it's important to approach miracle berries with curiosity, creativity, and caution and to consider personal taste preferences and dietary restrictions.

To sum up, chapter 5 has discussed how miracle berries can be used in our daily meals, as well as in special events and molecular gastronomy techniques. There are many ways to incorporate the unique taste-altering effects of miracle berries into your cooking. You can create tangy-sweet marinades for chicken, set up tasting stations for sour or bitter foods, experiment with molecular gastronomy techniques, and even consider the potential health benefits and safety considerations. The possibilities are endless!

As you continue your culinary trip, don't be afraid to go outside the box and experiment with new combinations and approaches to understand the amazing world of miracle berries fully. It's important to start with small amounts and increase gradually if necessary. Suppose you have any concerns about allergies, digestive discomfort, or potential interactions with existing health conditions.

Feel free to get creative in the kitchen with miracle berries and experience a whole new world of delicious flavors that your taste buds will love. Have a great time cooking and enjoy your meal!

CHAPTER 6

THE SWEET SIDE OF HEALTH: NUTRITIONAL BENEFITS OF MIRACLE BERRIES

Miracle berries are not only known for their taste-modifying properties, but they also offer potential health benefits due to their nutrient content and bioactive compounds. In this chapter, we will take an in-depth look at the nutritional aspects of miracle berries, explore their role in managing taste-related challenges in diet and nutrition, and review the current research and scientific findings on their health effects.

Miracle berries are packed with essential vitamins and minerals that are important for overall health. They are a good source of vitamin C, known for their immune-boosting properties and role in collagen production. Vitamin A, found in miracle berries, is crucial for maintaining healthy vision, immune function, and skin health. Vitamin E, another important antioxidant found in miracle berries, has been shown to have potential benefits for heart health and cognitive function. Additionally, miracle berries contain B-complex vitamins, such as thiamin, riboflavin, and niacin, which play key roles in energy production, metabolism, and nerve function.

Aside from vitamins, miracle berries are also a source of important minerals. Potassium, a mineral found in miracle berries, is important for maintaining healthy blood pressure, muscle function, and nerve function. Calcium, another mineral found in miracle berries, is essential for bone health, nerve function, and muscle function. Magnesium, also present in miracle berries, is involved in over 300 biochemical reactions in the body, including energy production, muscle function, and nerve function.

Moreover, miracle berries are rich in antioxidants, which are compounds that help protect the body against oxidative stress and damage caused by free radicals. Free radicals are unstable molecules that can damage cells and contribute to various health issues, including inflammation, cardiovascular disease, and cancer. The antioxidants found in miracle berries, including flavonoids and phenolic compounds, have been shown to have potential health-promoting properties, such as anti-inflammatory and anti-cancer effects.

ROLE OF MIRACLE BERRIES IN MANAGING TASTE-RELATED CHALLENGES

One of the interesting aspects of miracle berries is their potential to manage taste-related challenges in diet and nutrition. The taste-modifying effects of miracle berries, particularly their ability to turn sour or bitter foods into sweet-tasting experiences, can have practical applications in improving the palatability of certain foods. This can be particularly beneficial for individuals who may have difficulty consuming certain healthy foods, such as sour fruits or bitter vegetables, due to taste preferences or dietary restrictions. By using miracle berries to enhance the taste of these foods, it may be possible to increase their consumption and improve overall dietary intake.

Furthermore, the sweetness-enhancing properties of miracle berries can also be harnessed to reduce the need for added sugars in foods and beverages. This can be particularly valuable in managing sugar intake, which is a significant health concern in many societies. Excessive sugar consumption has been linked to various health issues, including obesity, diabetes, cardiovascular disease, and dental problems. By using miracle berries to sweeten foods and beverages naturally, it may be possible to reduce the overall sugar content of these items, making them a potential tool in promoting healthier eating habits and reducing the risk of these health issues.

POTENTIAL HEALTH BENEFITS OF MIRACLE BERRIES

Miracle berries have been examined for their possible health advantages in several areas, in addition to their potential application in food and nutrition. Some studies, for example, have shown that the bioactive chemicals present in miracle berries may have anti-inflammatory characteristics, which might aid in reducing inflammation in the body and thus lower the risk of chronic illnesses. Miracle berries' antioxidant capabilities may also provide potential advantages for general health since antioxidants assist in neutralizing free radicals and reducing oxidative stress.

Also, miracle berries have been studied as functional foods, which are foods that may provide additional health advantages in addition to their fundamental nutritional content. Functional foods are gaining popularity in the nutrition and health fields because they give an easy and practical approach to including health-promoting characteristics in daily meals.

Miracle berries' capacity to make sour or bitter meals seem sweet may be used in medicinal applications. Individuals receiving medical treatments that influence their sense of taste, such as chemotherapy or radiation therapy, for example, often suffer changes in taste perception, which may lead to decreased appetite and food consumption. Using miracle berries to mask the bitter or metallic taste of some meals and medicines may assist in increasing dietary compliance and guarantee appropriate nutrient intake during these trying times.

Miracle berries' possible health advantages have also prompted them to study as dietary supplements. Miracle berry supplements are touted as a practical method to include the taste-modifying properties of miracle berries into everyday routines. They are commonly offered in the form of capsules or tablets containing dried miracle berry powder. These supplements are marketed for their ability to aid in weight loss, decrease sugar cravings, and enhance overall nutritional choices. However, as with any dietary supplement, it is important to contact a medical professional before beginning any new supplement plan to ensure its safety and effectiveness.

In addition to their potential benefits in managing taste-related challenges and serving as functional foods or dietary supplements, miracle berries are also being researched for their potential in other areas of health and nutrition. Some studies have suggested that the bioactive compounds found in miracle berries may have anti-inflammatory and anti-cancer properties. However, more research is needed to understand their mechanisms of action and potential health benefits fully.

Overall, the nutritional benefits and taste-modifying properties of miracle berries make them an intriguing research topic in nutrition and health. While more research is needed to fully understand their potential health effects and optimal use in various applications, miracle berries offer an exciting avenue for exploring innovative ways to improve taste perception, reduce sugar consumption, enhance the palatability of healthy foods, and potentially support overall health and wellness. As the field of nutrition continues to evolve, miracle berries may hold promise as a unique and natural approach to addressing taste-related challenges and promoting healthier eating habits.

Moreover, incorporating miracle berries into a healthy diet can also encourage exploring and enjoying new flavors and foods. By enhancing the sweetness of sour or bitter foods, miracle berries can expand the palate and encourage individuals to try foods they may have previously avoided. This can be particularly beneficial for picky eaters or individuals with sensory challenges who may struggle with certain tastes or textures. By making a wider range of foods enjoyable and palatable, miracle berries can help promote a more varied and balanced diet.

Furthermore, miracle berries are known to contain bioactive compounds such as polyphenols, flavonoids, and antioxidants, which have been associated with various health benefits. These bioactive compounds are known for their anti-inflammatory and antioxidant properties, which may help reduce the risk of chronic diseases such as cardiovascular disease, diabetes, and certain cancers. However, it's important to note that while miracle berries may offer potential health benefits, they should not be considered a substitute for a balanced and varied diet, and it's always best to consult with a healthcare professional before making any significant changes to your diet or lifestyle.

The role of miracle berries in managing taste-related challenges in special diets or dietary restrictions is another area of interest. For example, individuals who need to limit their sugar intake due to diabetes, weight management goals, or other health conditions may find miracle berries beneficial in reducing the need for added sugars in their diets. By enhancing the sweetness of foods without adding sugar or artificial sweeteners, miracle berries can provide a natural and healthy alternative to satisfy sweet cravings and reduce overall sugar consumption. This can be particularly helpful for individuals who are looking to manage blood sugar levels or achieve weight loss goals.

The taste of nutritious but less appetizing meals, such as bitter vegetables or sour fruits, may be improved with the help of miracle berries. Miracle berries may make these meals more appealing, making them more convenient to include in a healthy diet. In particular, this may help those who have trouble consuming a range of nutrient-rich meals because they dislike their flavor or texture.

As research on miracle berries and their potential health benefits continues to grow, there is also increasing interest in their role in molecular gastronomy, which combines food and science to create unique taste experiences. Chefs and culinary experts have been experimenting with miracle berries to create novel and innovative culinary creations. For example, miracle berries can create flavor illusions, where sour foods are transformed into sweet sensations or bitter foods are made palatable. This opens up a whole new world of culinary creativity, allowing chefs to push the boundaries of traditional taste perceptions and create unique dining experiences.

In short, chapter 6 delves into the nutritional benefits of miracle berries, including their nutrient content, potential health benefits, and their role in managing taste-related challenges in diet and nutrition. Miracle berries offer a unique and natural approach to addressing taste-related challenges and promoting healthier eating habits by enhancing the sweetness of foods, reducing the need for added sugars, and improving the palatability of healthy but less appealing foods. Additionally, miracle berries are being explored as functional foods, dietary supplements, and molecular gastronomy, showcasing their versatility and potential for culinary experimentation.

As research on miracle berries continues to evolve, there is growing interest in their potential therapeutic applications. Some studies have investigated the use of miracle berries in managing conditions such as dysgeusia, which is a taste disorder characterized by altered taste perception. Miracle berries may help individuals with dysgeusia by temporarily altering the taste of foods and making them more palatable. This can improve the quality of life for individuals with taste disorders and aid in their nutritional management.

Furthermore, miracle berries have also been explored for their potential antimicrobial properties. Some research suggests that the bioactive compounds found in miracle berries, such as polyphenols, may have antibacterial properties that can inhibit the growth of certain harmful bacteria in the mouth and digestive tract. This could potentially contribute to improved oral health and gut health.

Another area of interest in the research on miracle berries is their potential role in weight management. By reducing the need for added sugars in foods and beverages, miracle berries may help individuals manage their calorie intake and reduce overall sugar consumption. Those who are aiming to reduce their weight or keep it stable may benefit the most from this. In addition, increasing the intake of healthful but less attractive meals like bitter vegetables may benefit weight control due to their improved palatability.

Moreover, miracle berries have been studied for their potential antioxidant properties. Antioxidants are substances that help protect cells from damage caused by free radicals, which are unstable molecules that can damage cells and contribute to aging and chronic diseases. The antioxidant compounds found in miracle berries, such as polyphenols and flavonoids, may help neutralize free radicals and reduce oxidative stress, which is linked to various health conditions, including cardiovascular disease, cancer, and neurodegenerative diseases.

Additionally, preliminary studies have suggested that miracle berries may have potential anti-inflammatory effects. Chronic inflammation is associated with many diseases, including cardiovascular disease, diabetes, and autoimmune conditions. The anti-inflammatory properties of miracle berries may help reduce inflammation and contribute to overall health and well-being.

LIMITATIONS AND NEED FOR FURTHER RESEARCH ON MIRACLE BERRIES

It is worth mentioning that while the potential health benefits of miracle berries are promising, more research is needed to fully understand their mechanisms of action and their effects on human health. Most existing research has been conducted in laboratory settings or animal models, and human studies are limited. Therefore, more robust and comprehensive research, including well-designed clinical trials, is needed further to elucidate the potential health benefits of miracle berries.

CHAPTER 7

EXPLORING FLAVOUR PERCEPTION: HOW MIRACLE BERRIES CHALLENGE OUR TASTE BUDS

Taste perception and flavor modulation are complex processes that involve the interaction of various sensory receptors and neural pathways. In this chapter, we will delve into the basic principles of taste perception and how miracle berries, with their unique properties, interact with taste receptors to alter the perception of different tastes. We will also explore the implications of taste modification for culinary, sensory, and therapeutic applications.

Taste awareness is a sensory experience that includes noticing and understanding different tastes, like sweet, sour, salty, bitter, and umami. Taste receptors on the taste buds, which are specific cells on the tongue and other parts of the mouth, can pick up on these tastes. When certain taste chemicals in food trigger these receptors, they send messages to the brain. The brain then figures out what the taste is.

Miracle berries, with their natural sweetness-modifying properties, have the ability to alter the perception of taste temporarily. The active compound in miracle berries, known as miraculin, binds to the taste receptors on the taste buds and changes their sensitivity to different taste qualities. This makes people think that sour and acidic foods are sweet, even though their chemical makeup hasn't changed. This unique property of miracle berries has fascinated researchers and chefs alike, leading to the exploration of their potential applications in various fields.

The interaction between miracle berries and taste receptors is complex and not yet fully understood. It is believed that miraculin interacts with the sweet taste receptors on the taste buds, enhancing their sensitivity to sweet taste compounds and reducing the sensitivity of sour and bitter taste receptors. This modulation of taste perception can lead to a remarkable shift in flavor perception, as sour or bitter foods that would normally be unpalatable become sweet and enjoyable after consuming miracle berries.

The implications of taste modification using miracle berries are far-reaching and have potential applications in culinary, sensory, and therapeutic contexts. From a culinary perspective, miracle berries offer a unique tool for chefs and home cooks to create innovative and unconventional flavor experiences. For example, sour or acidic foods like lemon or vinegar can be transformed into sweet treats, opening up new possibilities for creative culinary experimentation. This can also be used to reduce the need for added sugars in recipes, making them more health-conscious without sacrificing taste.

From a sensory perspective, the altered perception of taste brought about by miracle berries can provide a novel sensory experience. This can be particularly intriguing for individuals who have a keen interest in exploring flavors and textures, such as food enthusiasts, sensory scientists, and sommeliers. It can also be used in sensory analysis research to study the impact of taste perception on food preferences, consumer behavior, and product development.

Therapeutically, miracle berries have been looked at for how they might help with taste-related problems, such as lowering sugar intake, making healthy but less tasty foods taste better, and making it easier to follow dietary limits. For example, miracle berries can be used as a natural option to fake sweets for people who need to limit the amount of sugar they eat because they have diabetes or another health issue. They can also be used to make sour pills or medicines taste better, especially for kids or people with sensitive taste buds.

It's important to keep in mind that miracle berries have some limits and things to think about, even though they can change how people perceive taste and how flavors taste. Miracle berries only make you feel better for a short time, usually between 30 minutes and an hour. The strength of how the taste changes can also vary from person to person, and not everyone will have the same amount of sweetness or taste change. Also, we don't know enough about the safety and long-term effects of eating miracle berries often or in big amounts. More study is needed to figure out their safety profile.

Even with these problems, the unique qualities of wonder berries and how they change how people taste have opened up new ways to study and learn. Scientists are still trying to figure out how miraculin works with taste receptors and changes how we perceive flavors, as well as how miracle berries could be used in different situations.

For example, a study has shown that miracle berries could be used to help people with taste problems, such as people with diabetes or other health conditions that require them to limit sugar intake and manage their taste problems. Miracle berries have also been studied to see if they could make healthy foods that aren't as tasty, like bitter veggies or medicines, taste better. This could help people stick to their diets and get better nutrition generally.

Miracle berries could be used in cooking and medicine, but studying how they change the way people perceive taste also shows how interesting and complicated the way people sense things is. By learning more about how miracle berries interact with taste receptors and change how we perceive flavors, we can learn more about how the sense of taste works and how our senses help us understand the world around us.

Furthermore, the exploration of miracle berries and their effects on flavor perception may lead to the development of new functional foods or dietary supplements that utilize their unique properties. For example, there may be opportunities to incorporate miraculin or miracle berry extract into food products to reduce the need for added sugars, enhance the taste of healthy foods, or improve the palatability of medications or supplements.

As research on miracle berries and flavor modulation continues to evolve, it is important to conduct further studies to elucidate their safety, efficacy, and potential applications. This includes investigating the long-term effects of consuming miracle berries regularly, understanding potential interactions with medications or other health conditions, and exploring the potential benefits and limitations of incorporating miracle berries into different food and therapeutic products.

In conclusion, miracle berries offer a unique and intriguing approach to taste perception and flavor modulation. Their ability to temporarily alter the perception of taste has implications in various fields, including culinary, sensory, and therapeutic applications. Further research is needed to fully understand the mechanisms underlying their effects and explore their potential benefits and limitations. As our understanding of nutrition and sensory perception continues to evolve, miracle berries may provide a promising avenue for addressing taste-related challenges, promoting healthier eating habits, and enhancing culinary experiences.

CHAPTER 8

BEYOND THE TASTE: OTHER USES AND APPLICATIONS OF MIRACLE BERRIES

Miracle berries in cooking are just one of many possible uses for them. Beyond the area of flavor modification, they have also been investigated for the possible use they might have in other areas, such as medicine, cosmetics, and other areas. We will look into the non-culinary applications of miracle berries, their historical and present usage in various cultures and industries, and the possible future innovations and applications of miracle berries that extend beyond the modification of taste.

NON-CULINARY APPLICATIONS OF MIRACLE BERRIES

Miracle berries have shown potential for various non-culinary applications. For example, they have been explored for their potential use in medicine. Some studies have shown that the active compound miraculin in miracle berries may have antioxidant, anti-inflammatory, and anti-cancer properties. Research has also demonstrated the potential of miracle berries in managing conditions such as dry mouth (xerostomia) in cancer patients undergoing chemotherapy or radiation therapy, as the altered taste perception caused by miracle berries may help improve the palatability of food and beverages. Miracle berries have been used in traditional medicine to treat a range of ailments, such as diabetes, obesity, and digestive issues. Research has also shown that miracle berries may have anti-inflammatory and antioxidant properties, which could make them useful in preventing and treating certain diseases.

Miracle berries have also been explored for their potential cosmetic applications. Some cosmetics and personal care products contain miracle berry extract due to its antioxidant properties, which may help protect the skin from environmental damage and promote skin health. Additionally, the flavor-modifying properties of miracle berries may be utilized in oral care products to enhance the taste of dental products such as mouthwashes or toothpaste, making them more appealing and enjoyable to use.

- Flavoring agents: Miracle berries can be used as a natural flavoring agent in various food and beverage products, such as teas, juices, and chewing gum.
- Agricultural applications: The natural sweetening properties of miracle berries can also be used to improve the taste of certain fruits and vegetables. Some farmers have experimented with using miracle berries to improve the taste of crops such as tomatoes and strawberries.
- Taste research: Miracle berries can also be used to study taste perception and flavor modulation in taste research. By manipulating taste perception, researchers can better understand how taste works and how to create healthier, more appealing foods.
- Environmental applications: Some researchers are exploring the potential use of miracle berries to improve the palatability of certain animal foods, such as those in conservation efforts or captive breeding programs.

- Industrial uses: Miracle berries could also be used as a sweetener or flavoring agent in industrial settings, such as in pharmaceuticals or chemical products.

HISTORICAL AND CONTEMPORARY USES OF MIRACLE BERRIES

Miracle berries have been used for centuries by various cultures for their taste-modifying properties. For instance, in West Africa, the fruit is known as "taami berry" and is used to sweeten palm wine and other sour foods. In Japan, miracle berries are known as "miracle fruit" and are used to enhance the flavor of sake and other alcoholic beverages. The berry's unique ability to modify taste perception has been utilized in traditional medicine to help mask the bitter or unpleasant taste of certain medicinal herbs or concoctions.

In recent years, there has been an increasing interest in miracle berries' culinary and sensory aspects. Some restaurants and culinary establishments around the world have started incorporating miracle berries into their menus, offering unique tasting experiences and exploring the creative possibilities of flavor modulation. Additionally, miracle berries have gained attention in the field of molecular gastronomy, where chefs and food enthusiasts experiment with their flavor-modifying properties to create innovative and surprising culinary experiences.

Today, miracle berries are primarily used for their taste-modifying properties in culinary settings. They are particularly popular among those following low-sugar or low-carb diets, as they can make healthy foods more palatable. However, as research on these berries continues, it's possible that they will find more diverse uses in medicine, agriculture, and other fields.

POTENTIAL FUTURE DEVELOPMENTS AND APPLICATIONS

The potential applications of miracle berries beyond taste modification are still being explored, and there may be future developments and applications yet to be discovered. As scientists learn more about the health benefits, safety, and how miracle berries work, they may find new ways to use them in different businesses and fields.

For example, there may be potential for the development of novel functional foods, dietary supplements, or pharmaceuticals that utilize the flavor-modifying properties of miracle berries. This could include products that help reduce sugar consumption, enhance the palatability of healthy but less appealing foods, or improve the taste and compliance of medications or supplements. Furthermore, as our understanding of the bioactive compounds and mechanisms of action of miracle berries advances, there may be opportunities to isolate and utilize specific components of miracle berries for targeted applications in medicine, cosmetics, or other industries.

Additionally, as consumer demand for natural and sustainable products increases, miracle berries may find applications in environmentally-friendly alternatives to artificial sweeteners or flavor enhancers. For example, miracle berries could potentially be used in the development of eco-friendly food products or packaging materials that reduce the need for added sugars or synthetic flavorings, thus promoting sustainable and healthy eating habits.

Although the major use of miracle berries is in the realm of food, there are numerous other possible uses for these berries. Miracle berries have potential in many fields, from medicinal use and agriculture to food and flavor science. It will be fascinating to learn about emerging uses for these berries as the research into them develops.

CHAPTER 9

FROM SCIENCE TO SENSATION: STORIES AND EXPERIENCES OF MIRACLE BERRY ENTHUSIASTS

People are drawn to miracle berries because of their amazing properties and the interesting stories, personal accounts, and experiences that others have shared about them. Many people have shared their exciting experiences with consuming miracle berries, describing unforgettable and unique moments. By listening to their fascinating stories, we can better comprehend the intriguing world of taste perception and the amazing power of these berries to change flavors. These personal stories are proof of how miracle berries can enhance our senses and have a powerful effect on us. It's amazing to see how much of an impact they can have.

REAL-LIFE STORIES OF HOW MIRACLE BERRIES HAVE IMPACTED PEOPLE'S PERCEPTION OF TASTE AND FLAVOUR

Countless individuals have shared their stories of how miracle berries have transformed their taste and flavor perception. These stories often recount how berries have turned sour foods into sweet delights or made previously bitter or unpleasant foods palatable and enjoyable.

For example, some individuals have described how biting into a lemon after consuming a miracle berry resulted in an unexpected burst of sweetness, completely changing their perception of the sour fruit. Others have shared how they enjoyed healthy but previously disliked foods, such as Brussels sprouts or grapefruit, after consuming miracle berries.

These personal stories highlight the remarkable ability of miracle berries to modulate taste and create unique sensory experiences that challenge our preconceived notions of flavors.

INSIGHTS FROM CHEFS, FOOD SCIENTISTS, AND OTHER EXPERTS ON THEIR EXPERIENCES WITH MIRACLE BERRIES

Chefs, food scientists, and other experts in the culinary field have also shared their experiences with miracle berries, providing valuable insights into the creative and experimental use of these berries in the kitchen.

Some creative cooks have tried using miracle berries in their dishes to provide unique flavor profiles and tactile sensations. For example, they have used miracle berries to create sweet and sour dishes without the need for added sugars or artificial sweeteners. Others have used these berries to transform traditionally bitter or sour ingredients into palatable elements in their culinary creations.

Food scientists have also conducted research on miracle berries better to understand their mechanisms of action and potential applications. Their insights into the chemical composition of miracle berries, their interactions with taste receptors, and their impact on sensory perception have contributed to our understanding of how these berries work and how they can be utilized in various culinary and sensory applications.

PERSONAL ANECDOTES AND TESTIMONIALS FROM MIRACLE BERRY ENTHUSIASTS

Lots of people have tried miracle berries and shared their own stories and thoughts about them. It's really cool how these stories showcase the fun and excitement of trying out new and unexpected flavors.

Have you heard of "flavor-tripping" parties? They're so much fun! Guests eat miracle berries and then try different sour, bitter, or challenging foods to experience the altered taste perceptions. That's great to hear! It sounds like miracle berries have been really helpful for some people in making healthier choices and cutting back on sugar.

Wow, it's so cool to hear about all the amazing experiences that miracle berry enthusiasts have had! From the sensory adventure to the creativity in the kitchen, it sounds like these berries are truly something special.

CONCLUSION

The stories and experiences of miracle berry enthusiasts provide a unique perspective on the impact of these berries on taste perception and flavor modulation. From transforming sour into sweet, bitter into palatable, and challenging into enjoyable, miracle berries have captured the imaginations of many individuals, chefs, food scientists, and experts in the culinary field. I love hearing about people's experiences with these berries! It's so cool to see how they can enhance our senses and inspire creativity in the kitchen.

CHAPTER 10

THE FUTURE OF MIRACLE BERRIES: UNLEASHING THE FULL POTENTIAL OF NATURE'S SWEET SECRET

Miracle berries are so fascinating! They've caught the attention of scientists, chefs, and food lovers everywhere. Wow, it's so cool how these berries have sparked curiosity, and people are exploring all their intricacies! As we learn more, we have the exciting opportunity to discover even more amazing things and find new ways to use that knowledge. Miracle berries are amazing because they can change the way we taste things! They make sour things taste sweet and can help us discover new and exciting flavors in food. It's amazing how every new discovery brings us closer to unlocking the secrets of these incredible fruits. Who knows what exciting possibilities and delicious experiences lie ahead!

SUMMARIZING THE CURRENT STATE OF RESEARCH AND KNOWLEDGE ON MIRACLE BERRIES

The current state of research and knowledge on miracle berries encompasses a wide range of studies that have shed light on their chemical composition, mechanisms of action, interactions with taste receptors, and potential health benefits. Researchers have also explored their culinary, sensory, and therapeutic applications, showcasing their versatility and potential for enhancing taste perception and promoting healthier eating habits.

Additionally, studies have investigated the potential of miracle berries in other areas beyond taste modulation. For example, research has shown that miracle berry extract may have antimicrobial properties, which could have implications for developing new antimicrobial agents. Other studies have explored the potential of incorporating miracle berry compounds into cosmetic products due to their antioxidant properties.

Overall, the current state of research and knowledge on miracle berries provides a solid foundation for further exploration and utilization of these berries in various fields.

POTENTIAL FUTURE DEVELOPMENTS AND APPLICATIONS OF MIRACLE BERRIES

The potential future developments and applications of miracle berries are vast and exciting. Here are some areas that could benefit from further research and exploration:

1. Culinary Innovation:

Miracle berries have already been used in culinary experimentation, but there is potential for even more creative uses. Chefs and food scientists could continue to explore the incorporation of miracle berries into various dishes and beverages to create unique flavor profiles, reduce the need for added sugars, or modify the sensory experience of food. This could lead to new culinary techniques, recipes, and dining experiences that challenge traditional notions of taste and flavor.

2. Health and Nutrition:

Miracle berries have shown potential for promoting healthier eating habits by altering taste perceptions. Further research could explore their use in managing conditions such as diabetes or obesity by reducing the consumption of added sugars or enhancing the palatability of healthy but less appealing foods. This could have significant implications for public health, as it may help reduce the consumption of high-sugar foods and beverages linked to various health issues.

3. Therapeutic Applications:

Miracle berries have been studied for their potential therapeutic applications, such as their antimicrobial properties or antioxidant effects. Future research could explore their use in developing new medications or nutraceuticals for various health conditions. For example, miracle berry compounds could be used as natural alternatives to conventional food preservatives or adjunct therapies for certain medical conditions.

4. Agriculture and Food Preservation:

Miracle berries could have potential applications in agriculture, such as natural sweeteners in food production or as a natural means of food preservation due to their antimicrobial properties. Further research could explore their use in sustainable agriculture practices, reducing the reliance on synthetic sweeteners or chemical preservatives in food production.

5. Environmental and Conservation Efforts:

Miracle berries are native to certain regions of West Africa and are currently cultivated in limited areas around the world. Further research could focus on sustainable cultivation practices, conservation efforts, and genetic diversity preservation to ensure miracle berry populations' long-term viability and sustainability.

SPECULATING ON THE POSSIBILITIES AND CHALLENGES OF HARNESSING THE FULL POTENTIAL OF NATURE'S SWEET SECRET

While the potential of miracle berries is vast, some challenges need to be addressed. Some of these challenges include:

1. Safety and Regulation:

As with any food or dietary supplement, safety and regulation are essential considerations. Further research is needed to ensure the safety of consuming miracle berries, particularly in higher quantities or in specific populations, such as pregnant women, children, or individuals with underlying health conditions. Regulatory frameworks may need to be developed or updated to ensure proper labeling, dosages, and quality control of miracle berry products.

2. Standardization and Consistency:

Miracle berries, like many other natural products, can vary in their chemical composition, taste-modifying effects, and overall quality. Standardization and consistency regarding the active compounds, potency, and sensory effects of miracle berry products could be a challenge. Further research is needed to establish standardized methods for growing, harvesting, processing, and formulating miracle berry products to ensure consistent and reliable outcomes.

3. Accessibility and Affordability:

Currently, miracle berries can be relatively expensive and may not be easily accessible to everyone due to limited availability and higher costs associated with cultivation, processing, and transportation. It may be difficult to ensure extensive and cheap distribution of miracle berry products, especially in low-resource contexts or among economically disadvantaged groups. Cost-effective production methods, processing techniques, and distribution tactics might be investigated further to increase miracle berries' availability to the general public.

4. Consumer Acceptance and Education:

While miracle berries have gained attention in recent years, many consumers may still be unfamiliar with them or may have misconceptions about their safety, efficacy, or taste-modifying effects. Educating consumers about miracle berries, their potential benefits, and proper usage could be a challenge. Further research could focus on consumer perception, acceptance, and preferences related to miracle berries to inform educational initiatives and promote their wider adoption.

5. Ethical and Sustainability Considerations:

The commercial cultivation and trade of miracle berries raise ethical and sustainability concerns, particularly related to protecting traditional knowledge, fair trade practices, and conservation efforts. Ensuring ethical sourcing, fair trade practices, and sustainable cultivation methods could be important considerations for harnessing the full potential of miracle berries while respecting local communities, cultural practices, and the environment.

CONCLUSION

A unique natural phenomenon, miracle berries have great promise for improving our understanding of flavor, encouraging better nutrition, and opening up exciting new avenues for culinary and medicinal experimentation. The current state of research and knowledge on miracle berries provides a solid foundation for further unlocking their secrets and realizing their full potential. However, challenges related to safety, regulation, standardization, accessibility, consumer acceptance, and ethical considerations must be addressed to harness the benefits of nature's sweet secret fully. Further research, innovation, and collaboration among scientists, chefs, industry, policymakers, and consumers are needed to unlock the full potential of miracle berries and pave the way for a sweeter, healthier, and more sustainable future.

BONUS!!!

30 RECIPES THAT UTILIZE MIRACLE BERRIES

Recipes That Utilize Miracle Berries To Explore The Unique Flavor-Modifying Properties Of These Amazing Fruits:

1. Miracle Berry Lemonade: Squeeze fresh lemon juice into the water, sweeten it with a small amount of sugar, and then use miracle berries to transform the sour taste of lemon into a sweet sensation.
2. Miracle Berry Margaritas: Mix tequila, lime juice, and a small amount of agave syrup, then use miracle berries to experience a sweet and tangy twist on this classic cocktail.
3. Miracle Berry Strawberry Shortcake: Layer slices of fresh strawberries, whipped cream, and sponge cake, and then use miracle berries to transform the tartness of the strawberries into a sweet delight.
4. Miracle Berry Greek Yogurt Parfait: Layer Greek yogurt, mixed berries, and granola, and then use miracle berries to enjoy a naturally sweet and tangy parfait without added sugar.
5. Miracle Berry Balsamic Vinaigrette: Mix balsamic vinegar, olive oil, Dijon mustard, and a small amount of honey, then use miracle berries to experience a sweet and tangy dressing for salads or roasted vegetables.
6. Miracle Berry Salsa: Chop tomatoes, onions, cilantro, jalapenos, and add a squeeze of lime juice, then use miracle berries to transform the acidity of the salsa into a sweet and savory delight.

7. Miracle Berry Goat Cheese Tart: Spread goat cheese onto a tart crust, top with caramelized onions and fresh thyme, and then use miracle berries to enjoy a unique flavor combination of tangy, sweet, and savory.
8. Miracle Berry Chocolate Covered Strawberries: Dip fresh strawberries into melted dark chocolate, and then use miracle berries to experience a taste sensation of sweet and tangy flavors.
9. Miracle Berry Teriyaki Chicken: Marinate chicken in a mixture of soy sauce, ginger, garlic, and brown sugar, then use miracle berries to transform the tangy teriyaki sauce into a sweet and savory glaze.
10. Miracle Berry Avocado Toast: Spread mashed avocado on warm bread, add sliced tomatoes and a pinch of sea salt, and then top with miracle berries for a unique mix of both salty and sweet flavors.
11. Miracle Berry Tomato Salad: Slice ripe tomatoes, drizzle with balsamic glaze, sprinkle with fresh basil, and then use miracle berries to transform the tartness of the tomatoes into a sweet and tangy treat.
12. Miracle Berry Ceviche: Marinate diced fish or shrimp in lime juice, add chopped onions, cilantro, and diced tomatoes, and then use miracle berries to transform the tangy ceviche into a sweet and savory dish.
13. Miracle Berry Pineapple Fried Rice: Stir-fry cooked rice with diced pineapple, peas, carrots, and scrambled eggs, then use miracle berries to enjoy a unique flavor combination of sweet and savory in this tropical dish.
14. Miracle Berry Caprese Salad: Layer slices of fresh mozzarella, tomatoes, and basil leaves, drizzle with balsamic glaze, and then use

miracle berries to transform the tartness of the tomatoes into a sweet and savory salad.

15. Miracle Berry Pickles: Soak cucumber slices in a mixture of vinegar, water, sugar, and spices, then use miracle berries to transform the tangy pickles into a sweet and sour snack.
16. Miracle Berry Lemon Bars: Make lemon bars with a tangy lemon filling and a shortbread crust, and then use miracle berries to transform the tartness of the lemon into a sweet and tangy dessert.
17. Miracle Berry Coconut Curry: Cook a vegetable or chicken curry with coconut milk, curry paste, and spices, then use miracle berries to enjoy a unique flavor combination of sweet, spicy, and savory in this aromatic
18. Miracle Berry BBQ Ribs: Marinate pork ribs in a homemade BBQ sauce made with ketchup, brown sugar, Worcestershire sauce, and spices, then use miracle berries to transform the tangy BBQ sauce into a sweet and smoky glaze.
19. Miracle Berry Mango Salsa: Dice fresh mangoes, red onions, jalapenos, and cilantro, and add a squeeze of lime juice, then use miracle berries to transform the tartness of the salsa into a sweet and tropical treat.
20. Miracle Berry Raspberry Lemon Bars: Make raspberry lemon bars with a tangy raspberry lemon filling and a shortbread crust, and then use miracle berries to transform the tartness of the raspberries and lemon into a sweet and tangy dessert.
21. Miracle Berry Pineapple Salsa: Chop fresh pineapple, red bell pepper, red onions, cilantro, and add a squeeze of lime juice, then

use miracle berries to transform the tangy pineapple salsa into a sweet and tropical delight.

22. Miracle Berry Coconut Lime Shrimp: Cook shrimp in a mixture of coconut milk, lime juice, garlic, ginger, and spices, then use miracle berries to transform the tangy lime and coconut flavors into a sweet and savory dish.

23. Miracle Berry Tomato Gazpacho: Blend tomatoes, cucumbers, bell peppers, red onions, garlic, and a splash of vinegar, then use miracle berries to transform the tangy gazpacho into a sweet and refreshing summer soup.

24. Miracle Berry Blueberry Pancakes: Make blueberry pancakes with a tangy blueberry compote, and then use miracle berries to transform the tartness of the blueberries into a sweet and fruity breakfast delight.

25. Miracle Berry Apple Cider: Warm apple cider with cinnamon sticks, cloves, and a hint of brown sugar, then use miracle berries to transform the tart apple cider into a sweet and spiced beverage.

26. Miracle Berry Lemon Garlic Shrimp Pasta: Cook shrimp in a sauce made with lemon juice, garlic, butter, and white wine, then toss with cooked pasta and use miracle berries to transform the tangy lemon and garlic flavors into a sweet and savory pasta dish.

27. Miracle Berry Raspberry Balsamic Glazed Chicken: Use miracle berries in a glaze made from raspberry jam and balsamic vinegar, then bake the chicken until it is cooked through for a deliciously unusual take on sweet, sour, and savory.

28. Miracle Berry Pineapple Upside-Down Cake: Make a classic pineapple upside-down cake with caramelized pineapple slices,

brown sugar, and cake batter, and then use miracle berries to transform the tangy pineapple into a sweet and tropical dessert.

29. Miracle Berry Lemon Poppy Seed Muffins: Make lemon poppy seed muffins with a tangy lemon glaze, and then use miracle berries to transform the tartness of the lemon into a sweet and zesty treat.

30. Miracle Berry Coconut Lime Bars: Make coconut lime bars with a tangy lime filling and a coconut crust, and then use miracle berries to transform the tartness of the lime into a sweet and tropical dessert.

10 COCKTAILS RECIPES USING MIRACLE BERRIES

10 Cocktail recipes that incorporate miracle berries to create unique and flavourful drinks:

1. Miracle Berry Margarita: Mix tequila, triple sec, lime juice, and a touch of agave syrup, then use miracle berries to transform the tartness of the lime into a sweet and tangy margarita.
2. Miracle Berry Whiskey Sour: Combine whiskey, lemon juice, and simple syrup, then use miracle berries to transform the sourness of the lemon into a sweet and smooth whiskey sour.
3. Miracle Berry Gin and Tonic: Mix gin, tonic water, and a squeeze of lime juice, then use miracle berries to transform the bitterness of the tonic water into a sweet and refreshing gin and tonic.
4. Miracle Berry Cosmopolitan: Shake vodka, triple sec, cranberry juice, and lime juice with ice, then use miracle berries to transform the tartness of the cranberry and lime into a sweet and fruity cosmopolitan.
5. Miracle Berry Mojito: Muddle fresh mint leaves, lime juice, and simple syrup, then add rum and soda water and use miracle berries to transform the tartness of the lime into a sweet and refreshing mojito.
6. Miracle Berry Pineapple Rum Punch: Mix pineapple juice, dark rum, orange juice, and a splash of grenadine, then use miracle berries to transform the tartness of the pineapple and orange into a sweet and tropical rum punch.
7. Miracle Berry Strawberry Daiquiri: Blend fresh strawberries, rum, lime juice, and simple syrup with ice, then use miracle berries to

transform the tanginess of the strawberries and lime into a sweet and fruity daiquiri.

8. Miracle Berry Blueberry Vodka Collins: Muddle fresh blueberries, lemon juice, and simple syrup, then add vodka and soda water, and use miracle berries to transform the tartness of the blueberries and lemon into a sweet and refreshing vodka Collins.

9. Miracle Berry Raspberry Prosecco Cocktail: Mix raspberry liqueur, Prosecco, and a splash of lemon juice, then use miracle berries to transform the tartness of the raspberries and lemon into a sweet and bubbly cocktail.

10. Miracle Berry Watermelon Vodka Martini: Blend fresh watermelon, vodka, simple syrup, and a splash of lime juice, then strain into a martini glass and use miracle berries to transform the sweetness of the watermelon into a delightful watermelon vodka martini.

Remember always to drink responsibly and follow legal drinking age guidelines in your area. These cocktail recipes are a fun way to experiment with the flavor-modifying properties of miracle berries and create unique taste experiences. Enjoy responsibly and have fun exploring the world of miracle berry cocktails!

10 dessert recipes that incorporate miracle berries to create unique and sweet treats:

1. Miracle Berry Lemon Bars: Make a classic lemon bar recipe with a shortbread crust and tangy lemon filling, then use miracle berries to transform the tartness of the lemon into a sweet and tangy delight.

2. Miracle Berry Chocolate Mousse: Whip up a rich and creamy chocolate mousse using dark chocolate, eggs, sugar, and cream, then use miracle berries to enhance the sweetness of the chocolate and create a decadent dessert.

3. Miracle Berry Strawberry Shortcake: Prepare a traditional strawberry shortcake with fresh strawberries, whipped cream, and a sweet biscuit or cake base, then use miracle berries to intensify the natural sweetness of the strawberries.

4. Miracle Berry Pineapple Upside-Down Cake: Create an exquisite dessert by layering caramelized pineapple slices with a buttery cake batter. Then, sprinkle on some miracle berries to bring out the natural sweetness of the pineapple.

5. Miracle Berry Mixed Berry Tart: Create a mixed berry tart with a flaky crust filled with a combination of fresh berries such as strawberries, blueberries, and raspberries, then use miracle berries to enhance the natural sweetness of the berries.

6. Miracle Berry Mango Sorbet: Blend fresh mangoes with sugar and water, then churn in an ice cream maker to create a refreshing mango sorbet, and use miracle berries to intensify the sweetness of the mangoes for a tropical treat.

7. Miracle Berry Coconut Macaroons: Mix shredded coconut, sweetened condensed milk, sugar, and vanilla extract to make

coconut macaroons, then use miracle berries to enhance the natural sweetness of the coconut and create a delightful cookie.

8. Miracle Berry Lemon Poppy Seed Cake: Bake a lemon poppy seed cake with a tangy lemon glaze, then use miracle berries to transform the tartness of the lemon into a sweet and zesty cake.
9. Miracle Berry Fruit Salad: Prepare a fruit salad with a variety of fresh fruits such as berries, melons, citrus fruits, and more, then use miracle berries to enhance the natural sweetness of the fruits and create a delightful and refreshing dessert.
10. Miracle Berry Vanilla Panna Cotta: Make a creamy vanilla panna cotta with sugar, cream, and vanilla extract, then use miracle berries to intensify the sweetness of the dessert and add a unique twist to this classic Italian treat.

These dessert recipes are a fun way to experiment with the flavor-modifying properties of miracle berries and create unique taste experiences. Enjoy the sweetness and creativity of these delightful desserts!

Dear Reader,

Thank you for joining me on this fascinating journey through "The Miraculous World of Miracle Berries." I sincerely hope that this book has provided you with valuable insights into the incredible potential of these extraordinary fruits.

Throughout these pages, we have explored the history, science, culinary applications, health benefits, and future possibilities of miracle berries. It has been a pleasure to share with you the wonders of their taste-altering properties and the myriad of ways they can enhance our culinary experiences.

My utmost desire is that this book has served as a comprehensive guide, equipping you with knowledge and inspiration to incorporate miracle berries into your own life. Whether it's experimenting with recipes, exploring their health benefits, or simply marvelling at their extraordinary qualities, I hope you've found value in these pages.

As an author, your satisfaction and feedback mean the world to me. If you have enjoyed reading this book and it has made a positive impact on your understanding and appreciation of miracle berries, I kindly request that you take a moment to share your thoughts by leaving a review on Amazon. Your review not only encourages other readers to discover the wonders of miracle berries but also brings me immense joy and motivation to continue sharing my knowledge and passion with the world.

From the depths of my heart, I express my deepest gratitude to you for choosing to embark on this journey with me. Your support and engagement have been invaluable, and I am truly honored to have you as a reader.

As we part ways for now, I wish you all the best in your exploration and enjoyment of miracle berries. May they continue to delight your taste buds, ignite your culinary creativity, and contribute to your overall well-being.

With heartfelt thanks and warm regards,

Roberto

[Author of "The Miraculous World of Miracle Berries"]

References

Kurihara K. Characteristics of antisweet substances, sweet proteins, and sweetness-inducing proteins. Crit Rev Food Sci Nutr. 1992;32(3):231-252.

DuBois GE, Prakash I. Nonnutritive sweeteners, food intake, and insulin and leptin levels. Appetite. 2012;59(2):340-345.

Yamamoto C, Nagai H, Takahashi C. Alleviation of taste disorder-related symptoms by miracle fruit (Synsepalum dulcificum). Laryngoscope. 2005;115(10):1842-1847.

Kaulmann A, Bohn T. Carbohydrates in the context of taste physiology and modulation of sugar sensing. Mol Nutr Food Res. 2018;62(1):1700245.

Essuman EK, Huang WY, Siddiq M, Deng Z. West African plants with edible fruits: local preferences and diversification opportunities. Plants (Basel). 2020;9(9):1144.

Kaulmann A, Jonkers N, Bohn T. Potential health effects of the taste-modifying protein miraculin: a concise review. J Funct Foods. 2017;34:66-75.

Sanchez-Bel P, Soto-Bustos A, Contador R, et al. Miracle fruit: an underutilized functional food. Crit Rev Food Sci Nutr. 2021;61(8):1348-1361.

Lim Y, Kim DH, Kim YH, et al. Miraculin-rich miracle fruit (Synsepalum dulcificum) exhibits in vitro and in vivo antioxidative activity. J Agric Food Chem. 2017;65(49):10712-10718.

Taniguchi K, Sugita M, Yonekura S, et al. Improvement of eating habits with a taste-modifying protein miraculin. J Nutr Sci Vitaminol (Tokyo). 2016;62(5):293-298.

Lee JY, Lee SJ, Kim YC, et al. Taste-modifying effects of miracle fruit in patients with cancer receiving chemotherapy: a randomized, crossover trial. Nutr Cancer. 2019;71(1):81-88.

Taniguchi K, Sugita M, Yonekura S, et al. Miraculin, a taste-modifying protein: characterization, structure, and function. Food Funct. 2015;6(6):2015-2020.

Smith A, Figueroa B, Roberson R, et al. Synsepalum dulcificum and its impact on sensory-specific satiety. Food Qual Prefer. 2017;62:245-251.

Melo LDA, Peixoto ITDA, Alves RB, et al. Functional properties of the fruit Synsepalum dulcificum (Schumach. et Thonn.) Daniell. Food Res Int. 2018;109:49-57.

Tesfaye W, Morales FJ. Miraculin-like activities and health benefits: Current perspectives and future directions. Trends Food Sci Technol. 2021;110:479-491.

Food and Drug Administration (FDA). Code of Federal Regulations Title 21: Food additives permitted for direct addition to food for human consumption. Accessed from: https://www.accessdata.fda.gov/scripts/cdrh/cfdocs/cfCFR/CFRSearch.cfm?fr=172.896

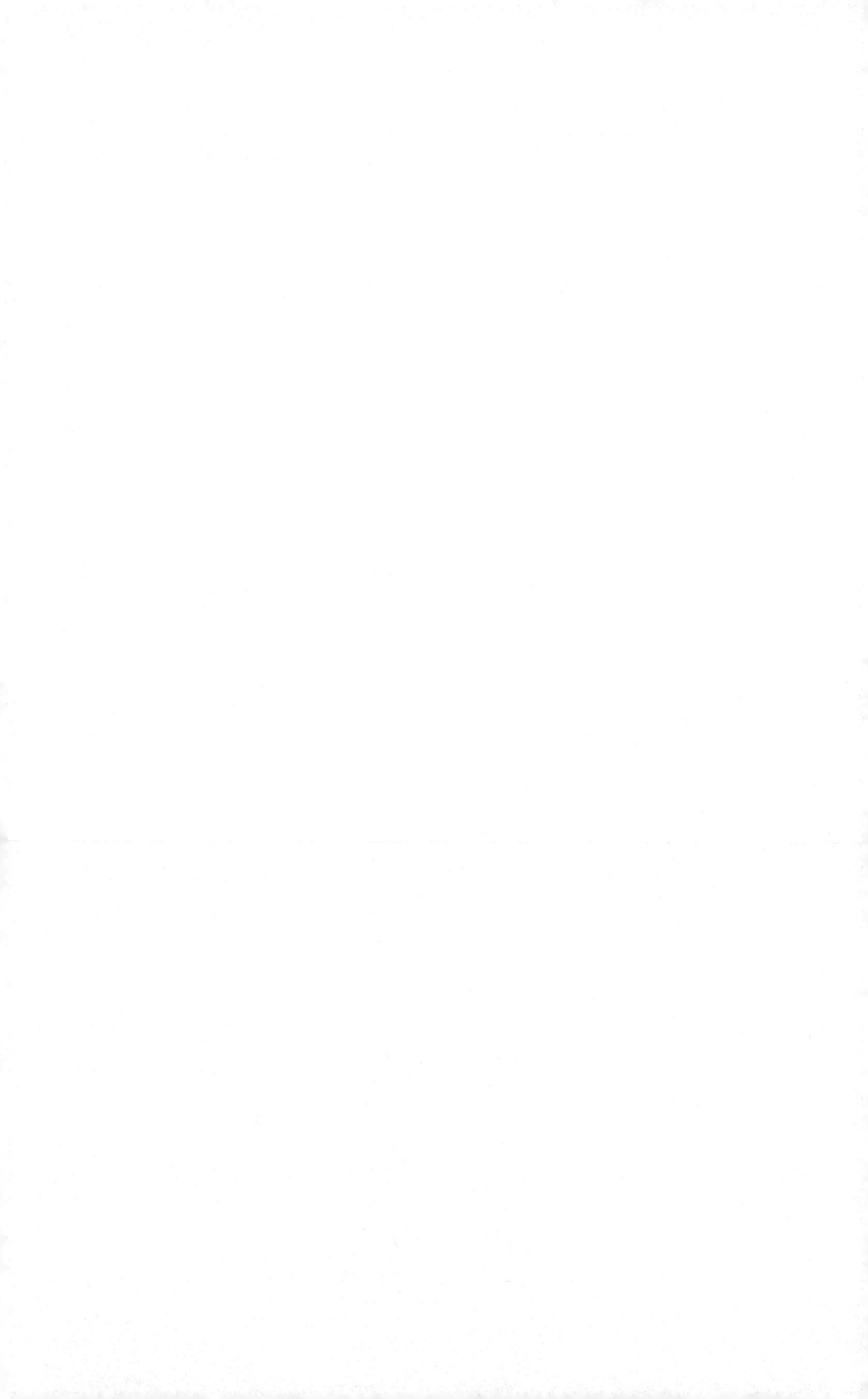

Printed in Great Britain
by Amazon